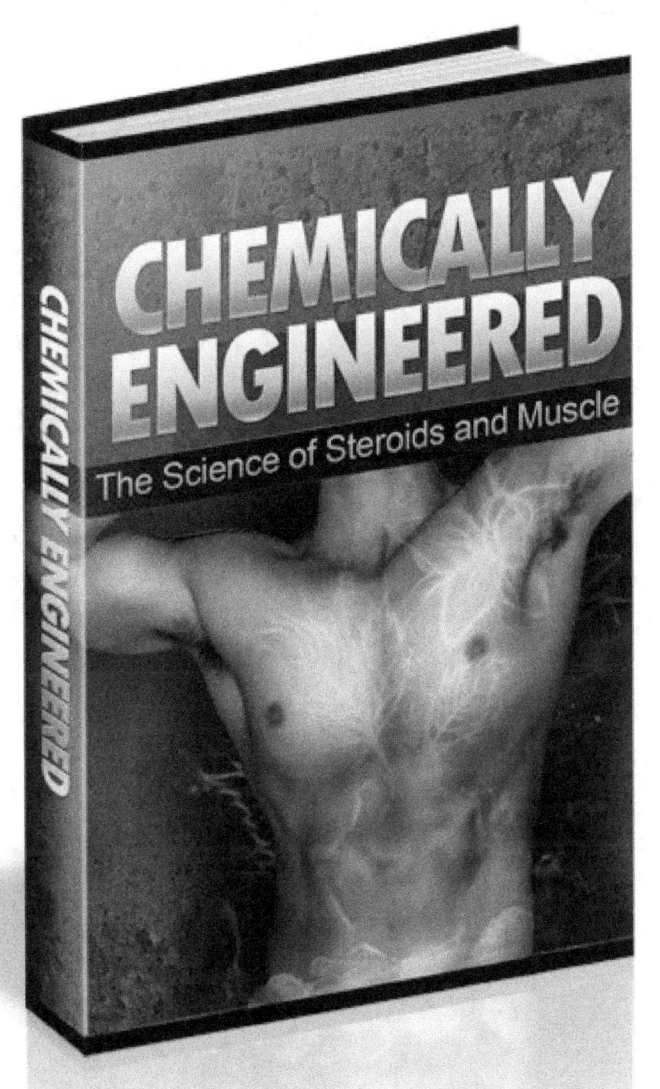

Table of Contents

Chapter 1 Be Smart

This guide is for those who are looking to educate themselves about steroids, and other performance enhancing drugs.

Even if you never intend to use steroids you will learn about how the chemicals in our bodies act in positive or negative ways on muscle growth.

If you are an experienced bodybuilder who feels that you have reached your genetic potential, and wish to exceed it then you have likely thought about steroids. By reading this guide you are obviously sensible and mature enough to educate yourself on how performance enhancing drugs work on the body.

Be Smart

Before we get into the discussion of steroids I am quickly

going to go over some important points.

1) Steroids need to be used carefully. These are powerful hormones and they are not without their dangers.

2) Steroids are not a magic pill. You need to eat, train, and rest.

3) Post cycle therapy is absolutely necessary.

Side effects of steroids and other performance enhancing drugs:

Acne, male pattern baldness, erectile disfunction, shrunken testicles, decreased sperm count, (Hypogonadism), breast tissue in males (Gynecomastia), liver damage, changes in cholesterol levels, stunted height, cardiovascular problems, enlarged prostate, water retention, depression, mood changes, and the shutting down of natural hormonal production.

Also in females side effects include menstrual changes, cervical cancer, virilization symptoms such as an enlarged clitoris, deepening of voice, and abnormal hair growth.

With Human Growth Hormone (HGH) use there is the added

increased risk of cancer and diabetes, joint swelling, joint pain, changes in bone structure, Acromegaly (Abnormal growth of organs), and body odor.

You should be at least 21 years of age before even considering altering your body chemistry. In youths steroids can have a negative effects on growth, and cause serious permanent side effects. Besides, when you are in your late teens and early twenties your body is naturally producing enough hormones to build and impressive physique.

It is not worth pumping your body full of chemicals in an attempt to create the kind of body that has been popularized in the media. The men and women you see in fitness magazines and in bodybuilding competitions with abnormally massive physiques often use excessive amounts of drugs to achieve that look.

Some bodybuilders take ten times the recommended dosages. This takes a serious toll on the body and also costs thousands of dollars to purchase the drugs. At that stage of the game steroids are definitely cause side effects. Then to off-set those side effects and in order to maintain a body chemistry that is fit for lean muscle growth more drugs have to be taken. Not only can this be unhealthy and expensive, but they also practically are walking chemistry sets.

There is a lot of knowledge that is required to use steroids safely and effectively while minimizing those side effects. A person should definitely not use steroids unless they are prescribed by a physician, or they have at the very least done their homework and understand how steroids act on the body.

You should have a solid base of bodybuilding, and weight lifting knowledge, and be in good physical condition with low body fat. If you are just starting out weight lifting give yourself a few years of training without steroids. If during this time you still wish to enhance yourself chemically learn everything you can about steroids and your bodies chemistry.

Obviously steroids do work. You can quickly pack on 15-20 pounds of muscle in a short amount of time on an initial cycle.

The body also quickly regulates itself making it more resistant to further cycles so higher doses will be required in the future to achieve the same effects. This is why steroids are taking in cycles that are commonly around 12 weeks on and then 12 weeks off. When off the cycle your body will no longer be producing as much testosterone as it did before you started your cycle. It takes time for your hormone levels to get back to normal. Post cycle therapy is used to get your body back on track while minimizing muscle loss, and side effects.

Don't think you can casually use steroids and not do post cycle therapy. In order to do steroids right you have to take care of your body when coming off of them. If you don't, your not being smart. If your not being smart then you shouldn't be using steroids at all.

Be sure you read this guide thoroughly, and refer to it often before, during, and after your cycle. It is recommended that you print out the charts, and quick start guides so you can have the information on hand and go through the material easily while taking notes.

When steroids are done right, along with a nutritious diet, intense weight training, and plenty of rest the results are spectacular. You can go beyond your genetic potential and build a body that is strong, with powerful lean muscle mass.

Chapter 2 Doing It Right

Do fool yourself into thinking it will be easy or effortless. Nothing worthwhile comes by taking shortcuts. You will need to train intensely, and progressively increase the amount of weight you lift. You will have to eat a healthy balanced diet that is rich in protein, healthy fats, carbs, and fiber. It will take a strong will, determination, focus, and dedication to lifetime of fitness.

Bodybuilding is a long term endeavor whether you use steroids or not. Take the time to master every aspect of building a strong healthy body. Your results will only be as good as your weakest link. If your nutrition, training is inadequate, or your not getting enough rest, your working against yourself.

Be smart and become the master of your body and mind so you can achieve your goals in every aspect of your life.

Life is about balance. Make sure you have a healthy balanced lifestyle. Enjoy yourself. Spend time with your friends and loved ones. Never stop learning. Keep developing new skills. Work hard. Save your money.

Always be grateful for what you have, and live in the moment. If you are not enjoying the journey, but always looking towards a future where you will be stronger, sexier, or wealthier, you are missing out on life altogether.

Your going to have your ups and downs, but be sure to find pleasure in everything you do, and be grateful for the life you have in every moment.

Chapter 3 Goal Setting

In order to be a high performer at anything you need to set goals and then take steps to achieve them. Before using steroids it would be helpful to have some targets measurements that you would like to hit.

Before you can set your targets you need to know where you currently stand. Record your weight, and find out what your body-fat percentage is at. Body-fat calipers are inexpensive to purchase and easy to use. Also take measurements of your neck, arms, chest, and waist, and legs.

Now set the goals you would like to achieve. It is a good idea to aim for the stars, but you also have to be realistic. You don't want to set your goals to low, but you also don't want to set them so high that you end up disappointed if you don't reach them. Your goals should be challenging though, and it is better to aim for the stars and land on the moon.

Examples of goals to work towards would be gaining 10 Kg in two months, reducing your body-fat percentage 4% in 6 weeks, or putting two inches on your arms in 90 days.

****

Chapter 4 Steroid Basics

Anabolic steroids are artificially produced drugs that mimic the effects of the male sex hormone- testosterone. They help in building cellular tissue (and hence, lean muscle mass) through increased protein synthesis. Anabolic steroids also have androgenic properties that result in the highlighting of male characteristics because of which their official name is Anabolic-Androgenic Steroids (AAS).

Some of the common effects of using anabolic steroids include an increase in muscle mass, lean mass, strength, development of vocal chords, growth of facial hair and in development of male sex features. Overuse and abuse, however, can spell doom and lead to acne, development of male breasts, increased aggression, a high blood pressure and an imbalance of sex hormones in the human body.

First synthesized in the 1930s, anabolics steroids have been used to therapeutically . While the main usage of steroids was to increase muscle and bone density, they have also been used to induce male puberty and to help in chronic waste and degradation brought about by diseases like aids and cancer.

Anabolic steroids have been recognized by the American Council of Sports Medicine as being responsible for the increase of muscle mass when combined with proper diet.

The council also recognizes that Anabolic Steroids can also lead to a boost in the performance of athletes when taken at the right time.

Due to these reasons, dope tests conducted on athletes test for permissible limits of these steroids in the athletes' bodies before allowing them to take part in international sporting events.

AAS also happen to be the most commonly found banned drug in athletes' bodies in all major international sporting events.

The usage of AAS has been banned in major international sporting events because of the considerable advantages they lend to the user over others - commonly considered as cheating.

There are, however, many countries in the world where AAS drugs are allowed to be used in a controlled environment. Such countries usually have black markets where these drugs are sold without prescription- something that has been a constant issue of worry for the policy makers and the regulatory authorities.

History of synthesized AAS:

It was in the late 19th century that medical use and synthesis of testicle extracts had begun. The studies on the strength increasing characteristics of testicle extract were still being pursued at that time.

The first documented isolation of testicle extracts can be dated back to the year 1931 when Adolf Butenandt, a scientist from Marburg, was able to extract about 15 mg of a substance called the androstenone from hundreds of liters of urine. This can be considered to be the first major event in the world of synthesis and extraction of steroids.

Later, as time passed, mutually competing pharmaceutical firms from the Netherlands, Germany and Switzerland were heavily funding scientists and researchers to extract testosterone- a more powerful male hormone existent in the testes.

It was in 1935 that three scientists- Karoly Gyula David, E. Dingemanse, J. Freud and Ernst Laqueur were able to lay down the exact steps of synthesizing and isolating the much revered male hormone (which they later named testosterone).

The chemical method to prepare testosterone from cholesterol was established and formalized in August 1935 by another group of scientists. There were a couple of other methods used, and discoveries made in this direction by scientists from all over Europe. The Nobel Prize in Chemistry was given away to Butenandt and Ruzicka in 1939 for their work in this field.

Chemical synthesis of AAS:

It was in the 1940s the Eastern block countries and the Soviet Union started working on development of steroids to bring about enhanced performance in their athletes and to give them a certain advantage over the competition.

This showed results and soon the Soviet athletes were ruling the Olympic standings. Noticing the sudden increase in efficiency, lifting power and strength of Russian athletes, the Americans also started working on development of synthetic steroids to boost their chances at the Olympics. It was under the direction of American Chemist Dr. John Zeigler that the world saw the development of a strong anabolic steroid with low androgenic effects.

The composition was marketed as Dianabol and was an instant success in the commercial market. The FDA gave a nod to the drug and the steroid was used as a cure for burn victims and the elderly people who required to put on weight. It was around that time that the mass gaining effects of this wonder drug were being discovered and soon the drug was a hit in the underground market. The drug was used mostly by body builder and weight lifters without proper medical guidance and this often led to havoc. The abusers soon started witnessing effects like enlarged prostates, reduced testicles and other common steroid side effects.

Looking at the immense popularity and the negative effects it brought about on the amateur users, the IOC banned AAS in 1976. It was in the 1980s that the IOC decided a strict "out-of-competition" rule against athletes found to have used AAS even during their training period. This saw some awareness and sanity towards steroid usage even amongst the amateur users and normalized the usage to manageable proportion. This era saw the use of certified steroids rolling into the market and drug laws being enforced more stringently against steroid use and abuse.

Chapter 5 Steroid Metabolism

The term used to signify the complete set of reactions in the organisms producing or consuming steroids is called steroid metabolism.

Steroids include testosterone, estrogen, progesterone and cortisol. While testosterone is the male hormone and is naturally made in the male testes, progesterone and estrogen are made up in the placenta and the ovary- the female sex glands.

Testosterone is converted into progesterone and estrogen on the fly in both the males and females in order to regulate the balance of the respective hormones in the body.

There are certain enzymes and reactions in the nervous system that bring these changes about and artificial steroids increase the levels of hormones in the body- thereby bringing exaggerated effects. Steroid Metabolism is broadly divided into three phases namely synthesis, genesis and degradation.

Steroid Synthesis:

This is the process of producing or manufacturing steroids using simpler substances or precursors. Technically speaking, this is an anabolic metabolic process and results in creation of a pathway for the synthesis and production of steroids.

There are different pathways created in different organisms and in the case of human beings, it is the Mevalonate Pathway where the synthesis starts out from.

Steroidogenesis:

This is the process in which steroids are produced from cholesterol. The term also encompasses the process in which the first level steroids manufactured from cholesterol are transformed into other types of steroids.

The main products of steroidogenesis include androgens (testosterone), corticoids (aldosterone, cortisol), estrogen and progesterone. It would be worth noting that this is almost an exhaustive list of steroids that might actually be of importance to human beings and therefore, this is one of the most important steps of steroid metabolism.

Elimination of steroids:

This is the final step of steroid metabolism and is one of the most important processes. The elimination of steroids is very important from the body in order to maintain hormonal balance.

Scientifically, the steroid rings are typically oxidized by cytochrome oxidase enzyme which weaken the steroid ring. The weakening of the steroid ring helps the other enzymes into breaking up the steroid structure to form bile acids as the end products. These bile acids are handled by the liver and are secreted out in the bile- thus ensuring that the body is clear of the end products.

How they act:

There are three main ways of administering steroids into the body- oral tablets, skin patches, and by injection.

Although oral administration of steroids is the easiest, the testosterone that is actually used up at the end of the dosage is just about 1/6th the administered levels. This is due to the fact that the steroids are rapidly absorbed when taken orally and are then converted into useless metabolites. These are not only useless, but sufficiently difficult for the liver to break down. Thus, the intake has to be low- which means that even lower volumes of testosterone are actually available to act on the body.

Skin patches are also available to provide doses of the hormone to the bloodstream at a steady pace. Because oral administration can lead to liver damage over a period of time intermuscular injections are the most preferred way of using steroids. When steroids are injected they bypass the liver which is easier on the body.

Steroids act by penetrating the membrane of the cells they are supposed to act on. After this penetration is through, the steroids cling themselves onto the anabolic receptors of the cells. These receptors are located in the cytoplasm (one of the main areas of the cell body) of the cell. After this, the substance diffuses into the nucleus of the cell.

The nucleus is the center of activity in the smallest part of an organism- the cell. After entering the nucleus, the steroids start acting on the cell and bring about hormonal changes that are responsible for bringing about the desired changes- weight gain and increase in the lean muscle mass.

Steroids are known to bring about the increase in muscle mass in two ways - first up, they increase the synthesis of protein in the body and secondly, they inhibit the tiring up of the muscles (a process otherwise termed as catabolism- the reverse of metabolism).

An increased protein synthesis helps the body in gaining weight and also supplies the body with additional energy and strength to workout without tiring.

The inhibition of catabolism further inhibits the production cortisol- the stress hormone of the human body. This leads to the body being less fatigued during workout- which results in a more stringent workout combined with aggressive energy.

Some AAS have also known to increase the BMR (or the Basal metabolic rate) which greatly reduces the fat content of the body- thereby making more room for the muscles to expand. This explains as to why the use of steroids leads to a lean muscle mass increase.

Chapter 6
Effects Of Using AAS
(Anabolic Androgenic Steroids)

The effects of using Anabolic Androgenic steroids can be best understood if we take a look at the anabolic as well as the androgenic aspects of the drugs independently.

The effects of using AAS can be both separate as well as overlapping. We will take a look at each of these aspects through this chapter. Taken literally, the term anabolic signifies cell growth and the word androgenic refers to the maintenance of muscular characteristics.

Anabolic Effects:

Most of the effects for which steroids have found usage and gained popularity amongst bodybuilders and athletes account for the anabolic effects of steroids. The effects include increased muscle mass owing the heightened protein synthesis by way of amino acids, stimulation of bone marrow- leading to an increase in the RBC (Red Blood Cell) count in the body, a better bone profiling and an increased appetite. There are a number of processes (some of which we have discussed in the previous chapters) that lead to a step by step increase in the muscle mass of the body-thus leading to an increased muscular profile and strength over a period of time.

Androgenic Effects:

Androgenic effects of steroids are mostly centered around bringing about changes in the sex hormones of the human body.

Androgenic changes are responsible for the growth of clitoris in females and penis in male children, and increased libido, an increased urge to engage in coitus, increase aggression, growth of hair in the pubis region and well as facial hair, deepening of voice due to development of vocal cords, a decrease in the production of natural sex hormones (which is the body's way of controlling the hormonal count and maintaining the balance in the body) and a reduction in productions of sperm in the male.

The androgenic anabolic ratio of an AAS:

The preferred choice for bodybuilders would be a low androgenic : anabolic ratio. Some drugs have a high ratio and are recommended for use in androgen-replacement therapies in male.

Steroids with a lower ratio are considered therapeutically well suited to treating those with a anemia and osteoporosis. In effect, however, there are very low digressions in the way a substance with low ratio acts on the human body as compared to a substance with a high ratio. Still, to be on better grounds, a substance with a low ratio is always considered to be a safer bet.

The weight gaining effects of steroids have closely been studied over the last three odd decades and it has been determined that short term AAS use can result in up to 2 to 5 Kgs of weight gain in a short span of 10 weeks.

In some cases, the fat percentage was also seen to have been reduced while lean muscle mass increased. It has also been observed that the upper body is more prone to mass gain as compared to other parts of the body. The reason can be attributed to the fact that the upper body (neck, thorax, shoulders and arms) has the maximum number of androgen receptors in the body- which gives the desired effect at these areas.

The overall strength of the users is also seen to increase to about 15% to 25% of the baseline strength before the administering of drugs.

This increase, however, is dependent upon the amount of dosage and the kind of steroid being taken. Besides, the increase in strength is prominently more amongst regular bodybuilders and weightlifters as compared to those who'd have recently started weight training.

Adverse and psychiatric effects of steroid usage:

Some of the most common side effects of excessive steroid usage include loss of hair in men (due to conversion of testosterone to DHT), deepening of vocal chords and development of facial hair on females, gynecomastia (development of breast tissue in males), variation in the natural levels of cholesterol in the human body- which can lead to cardiovascular diseases, heart seizure and other coronary artery diseases.

Apart from these side effects, steroids simulate the sebaceous glands, which can lead to acne and other skin conditions. Oral anabolic steroids need to be burnt down and digested by the body and this can also lead to severe liver damage if the doses are not controlled or backed up by injections.

Excessive steroid usage can also lead to lack of interest in sexual activity as well as temporary or permanent infertility in case of males.

In short, excessive steroid use can really tamper with the hormonal balance of the body; something that is capable of leading one onto quite a lot of complications.

The negative effects on natural testosterone production due to over-use of steroids is magnified in during adolescence. It can lead to premature stoppage of bone growth, premature puberty and certain other conditions that can really affect the overall body structure of the user. It is for this reason that it is highly recommended that *people under 21 years of age should not use steroids*, and even if they do- it should be under proper medical assistance.

Psychiatric effects:

There have been documented case studies which prove that steroids abuse can use to maniac-like conditions often leading to aggression, hypertension and even suicide in some extreme cases.

Prolonged usage can cause withdrawal effects and a dependency on steroids. Because of excess testosterone and then withdrawl after a cycle there can be mood swings and heightened irritability. The term coined for describing this condition is popularly called as "roid rage" in common language and has been termed as "hypomania" by scientists and psychiatrists alike.

Chapter 7
Usage And Legal Use/Abuse of AAS

Almost all the major sporting organizations around the globe have banned the use of AAS- during tournaments as well as before or after them. Some of the most important organizations that have passed the verdict against AAS use include the International Olympic committee, FIFA, ITF, European Athletic Association, WWE and International Cricket Council.

In the US, Anabolic Steroids are listed as schedule 3 drugs and thus, having possession or using them without a prescription is deemed illegal.

It is only under controlled environment and with proper medical reasoning and backing that AAS can be used in the US.

In countries like the UK and Canada, similar restrictions exist on the usage and possession of AAS. In Canada possessing AAS might not land you in jail, but unprescribed usage, trading and export/import of these drugs will definitely get you into trouble.

In most of the countries around the world, AAS is banned and categorized at a minimum of schedule 4 while in some countries like Thailand or Mexico, these drugs are readily available and there are no restrictions whatsoever on their usage.

In the US, the movement against the abuse of AAS in sports had gathered pace after the controversial victory that Ben Johnson had got in the 1988 summer Olympics in Seoul.

The US Congress was adamant on listing the AAS as schedule three but the three major medical bodies of that time- American Medical Association, the FDA and the Drug Enforcement Administration supported the view that AAS should not be banned since the hormones are natural and therfore did not produce dependence in the long run. The addiction factor was considered to be absent. Nevertheless, these drugs were eventually banned because they were considered as giving the users an undue advantage over their competition and thus it was considered cheating.

Detection of steroids is usually carried out using urine samples and hair samples. Traces can also be found in blood and perspiration.

Depending upon the route of administration, the dosage and the substance used, anabolic steroids may be detected in the urine samples for a period lasting up to 30 days from the last usage. The detection of steroids is not an easy task and the metabolic compositions of a number of substances might actually overlap with those of endogenous steroids- often leading to confusion about the actual use and dosage of the substance.

Chapter 8 Steroid Cycles For Beginners

The biggest myth about bodybuilding and using steroids is that people feel whoever uses steroids will bulk up in the right proportions at the right places- this is a potentially dangerous myth.

Steroids are not magic and getting results ultimately rests in the hands of the users themselves. For a novice, getting confused is very easy since there is such a lot of information available all around.

In this part of the e-book, we will go over the basics of steroid usage to get maximum results. Improper use of steroids can cause serious problems. It is up to the user to be educated enough to use them the right way.

In this section of the e-book, we would be taking a look at a dummy cycle. Users are expected to make notes from this dummy cycle and apply them to whatever drugs they are using in the correct proportions. We are using the basic doses here and as a tip, we would like novice users to stick to the basic doses rather than trying out complicated ones. Cycles should be cost and health effective. After all, your main purpose of body building should be to become healthier, and not just build muscle and strength.

For beginners, we would start off with a 12 month cycle and this is most effective time period to use steroids for.

You are bound to experience a good amount of weight gain in the first month or so, but this will start to subside towards the end of the cycle.

At the beginning of your first cycle there will be significant effects on your body and you might experience side effects like acne and aggression.

Stick to the prescribed quantity and do not over-do these drugs.

The brief break up of the cycles is given below. Please note that we are looking at stacking here and in case you are not sure about your medical history, consult a doctor before trying this yourself. The break up of weekly dosage is as follows:

Testosterone- 400 mg per week for 12 weeks coupled with 20 mg/day of Dianabol for the first five weeks.

Stacking is optional and if you are not sure about your stacking potential and/or if you feel that the gains and the effects are too much for you to handle- keep off stacking and cut down on Dianabol doses. You can also eliminate Dianabol altogether if you are not being able to handle the effects well.

Testosterone form the base of any beginners cycle and this is a great substance for single use as well as for the purpose of stacking. Being a natural hormone, it'll bring upon positive changes to the body including the production and synthesis of protein and IGF. This leads to increased muscle mass and the hormonal changes bring about an increase in strength as well as aggressiveness in the gym.

There can be other medications that can be added to the dosage in case side effects persist. The chances of side effects showing up are very low at this dosage, but sore nipples and hair loss can be a concern for some people. In case of sore nipples, you can add 10 MG dosage of Nolvadex till the soreness subsides. Hair loss can be countered by using common medicated shampoos like nizoral and propecia.

Testosterone finally converts into two androgens- the DHT and the female hormone estrogen. Therefore, overdoing the dosage can really results in your body loosing its state of homeostasis- be careful and be considerate of the fact that hormonal imbalances can lead to irreversible changes over a period of time. The 400 mg dosage that we are talking about here should be administered through injections.

The other drug we are taking into perspective is Dianabol. Dianabol is also a testosterone based drug which is tweaked to be administered orally and the conversion of testosterone to androgens is highly limited in case of Dianabol.

Stacking this drug with injection based testosterone during the beginner cycle will help you rake in better gains and more strength during the initial few weeks of your cycle. This will also give your body the much needed testosterone with a highly subsidized rate of conversion to estrogen- thus making sure that the gains are prolonged and the aggression doesn't burn you out sooner than required.

Dianabol should never be used as a substitute for injection based testosterone at any cost since an oral dose of the injectible equivalent can actually do a ton of harm to your liver and kidneys since oral doses need to be broken up by the digestive system.

Another word of caution for those who are looking to follow this or related beginner steroid cycles- keep doing cardiovascular exercise for about 15 minutes each day- four times a week while on the cycle. The reason is simple- you can expect a weight gain of about 20 pounds or even more while on this cycle and the body needs to get used to the excess weight.

Make sure your heart and cardiovascular organs are responding well and that you are able to carry out regular day to day work with efficacy. Besides, some people might develop a "bloated" look. Most of it would be water retention and having a balanced diet during the cycle is very important to prevent that boating of the body.

The body needs to come out more chiseled and better toned than what it was before putting yourself on the cycle- thus apart from putting your body through immense workout routines and steroid usage, make sure you are taking a proper high-calorie, well balanced diet.

Chapter 9   Steroid Profiles

Dianabol

Dianabol is the brand name for Methandrostenolone. Dianabol is know as a very effective mass builder. Generally Dianabol is taken in a bulk cycle. Stacks well with Deca-Durabolin and Testosterone Enanthate.

Dianabol can have significant negative effects on the liver so cycles are normally no longer than 8 weeks.

The half life of Dianabol is about 4 hours. If you want to keep your blood level steady it is advised to take it throughout the day. You can also take it as a single dose which will give you a higher blood level at one time

Because Dianabol is a powerful steroid it comes with negative side effects. It converts to estrogen which can cause Gynecomastia. Nolvadex and/or Provironum can be taken as anti estrogens to combat this. Bloating is a huge problem, as you get a lot of water retention.

Cycle: Bulking

Half life: 4 hours
Active life: 8 hours
Aromatization: yes
DHT Conversion: no
Post Cycle Therapy: Clomid, Nolvadex, HCG

Winstrol

Winstrol is a brand name that Wintrhrop Labs gave for Stanozolol, which they developed in 1962. Stanozolol is a derivative of dihydrotestosterone.

However Stanozolol is not as strong as dihydrotestosterone. In fact Stanozolols anabolic properties are mild when compared to most compounds that are stronger. This being said Stanozolol is still a very good at building lean muscle. Its anabolic properties could even be compared to Dianabol, but Winstrol does not cause a person retain water like Dianabol does.

The muscle you gain while on Stanozolol is of higher quality when compared to other more estrogenic steroids.

One of the most favorable aspects of Stanzolol is that it doesn't convert to estrogen, so you don't need to use an anti-estrogen.

Because Stanozolol does not convert into estrogen there is no water retention. Instead of that puffy, bulky look that users end up with while bulking and on a steroid such as Dianabol you instead get a dry look, with lean looking muscle. For this reason it is often used during cut cycles, and is also very popular with runners. In fact Stanozolol is compound that Ben Johnson tested positive after becoming the worlds fastest man and winning the Gold in the 1988 Summer Olympics.

Stanzolol comes in tablet form, or liquid. The injectable liquid varies from other steroids in that it is suspended in water and not oil. You can easily identify Stanzolol by its white milky color.

It is common to stack Stanzolol with other steroids to increase its effectiveness. When bulking stack stanzolol with Testosterone, Dianabol, or Anadrol. A stack such as this will give the user good muscle gains, without having excessive amounts of water retention.

When using Stanzolol in a cutting stack it can be taken with Trenbolone. A stack such as this should give the user a ripped look. For those who are sensitive to gynecamastia Primobolan, Deca-Durabolin or Boldenone can be used.

Anavar

Anavar is the brand name for the anabolic steroid Oxandrolone. It was purposely designed to be mildly anabolic, so it could be used to safely stimulate growth in children.

Like Winstrol Oxandrolone is a derivative of Dihydrotestosterone. It also does not convert into estrogen. Excess estrogen limits linear growth, which explains why women stop growing before men, and why they are shorter in stature.

For bodybuilders Oxandrolone is most often used during cutting cycles. It can be combined with Primobolan or Winstrol to create hard looking muscle with good definition. Stronger androgens that do not aromatize such as Provironum or Trenbolone can be added to harden up the muscle while also making it easier to lose fat.

In a bulk cycle add Testosterone or Dianabol. The combination creates good strength gains along with higher quality muscle without the puffy look.

For women or those sensitive to side effects of more anabolic compounds stack Anavar with Winstrol, Primobolan, or Deca Durabolin. This combination should creates faster gains, but it also increases androgenic buildup.

Because Oxandrolone does not convert to estrogen there in no need to use anti-estrogens. In low dosages this steroid has only a small effect on natural testosterone production. In higher doses there are the usual side effects associated with steroids such as acne, male pattern baldness, and liver stress.

Androlic

Androlic is the brand name for Oxymetholone. While there are injectable versions of this steroid they are rare; oral Oxymetholone is far more common.

Androlic is believed to be the most powerful steroid available. It is similar to Dianabol in that you get massive gains in short periods of time.

You also get a lot of water retention with this steroid not because it aromatizes. In fact Androlic does not convert to estrogen so how it can cause Gynecomastia is a bit of a mystery.

Some people believe it is because Androlic acts directly on

estrogen receptors. There is no evidence to back this up thus further research is required before it is known how it can cause Gynecomastia.

Not everyone will experience gyno from Androlic, but approximately fifty percent of users might get this side effect. The use of an anti-estrogen while on a steroid cycle will effectively prevent Gynecomastia.

Mesterolone

Mesterolone is a oral steroid that is commonly sold under the brand name Provironum.

For the most part mesterolone is used to boost the libido or to treat other hormonal conditions. Even though it is a strong androgen its effect on body in terms of protein synthesis and muscle building is limited.

Mesterolone prevents steroids from from converting into estrogen, and for this reason it is used by bodybuilders to avoid gynecomastia. Unlike most oral steroids Mesterolone is easy on the liver.

Mesterolone is popular during the cut cycle. When using Winstrol, Anavar, or Primobolan by themselves there is very little androgenic content. By adding Mesterolone it raises the androgen levels, while reducing estrogen which leads to muscle hardening.

Usually small quantities can be taken even by female athletes, but it is an androgen and thus can cause virilization. Women should limit their dosage of Mesterolone to 25 mg, and keep they cycle short; no longer than four to five weeks. This small dose is helpful for women during the cutting phase as it helps harden up muscles, and makes it easier to burn body fat.

Deca

Deca durabolin or simply 'Deca' is a common brand name for the compound 'Nandrolone Decanoate'.

Deca happens to be the most commonly used and widely trusted anabolic steroid of all times.

The greatest thing about this drug is its efficiency; a small dose of 200-400mg per week is enough to give the desired results. The compound is called a bulking agent, due to the fast results it shows.

Normally, a user on Deca starts experiencing weight gain within 24 to 36 hours. The mass gain can be as high as 20 pounds in just one month, not to forget the extreme physical strength achieved. Due to this and many other reasons, Deca is used by body builders across the world.

Mode of Operation: The secret of Deca's fast results lies in its chemical structure. Its chemical composition is very similar to testosterone. However, unlike testosterone, Deca is not broken down into lower metabolite. This metabolite has far lesser side effects than any other anabolic steroid.

Advantages: Following are few of the many advantages of Deca over other steroids:

- Retains nitrogen in the body, resulting in muscular growth.
- Deca is silent in skin, scalp and prostate; therefore, those parts are completely safe from any side effect.
- It binds better with the muscle tissues. This results in a faster muscular growth than usual.
- It has few androgenic effects on the body.
- Very little side effects and in case adverse side effects occur they aren't very harsh. Although, it is said that adverse effects do not occur unless the steroid is misused.
- Increase in lean body weight with little dosage.
- Stays in the body over an administrable amount, for a year or so.
- Beneficial for body's defense mechanism.
- During HIV, it helps weak patients gain the required amount

of weight quickly.
- Increases stamina and endurance.
- Equally good for both men and women.

Disadvantages: Apart from all the pros of Deca, it has a number of mild side effects:

- Acne
- High Blood pressure
- Headache
- Nausea
- Peptic ulcer
- Edema
- Insomnia
- Hyper excitation
- Longer time needed for blood clot
- Shivering
- Diarrhea

All in all, Deca is an extremely powerful anabolic steroid, but it can also quickly shut down your natural testosterone production. For this reason Deca should mainly be used as a "secret weapon" to burst past plateaus that have been difficult to overcome.

Boldenone

Boldenone is an anabolic steroid sold under a variety of names like Equipoise, Ganabol and Ultragan. It is a man-made steroid having structure similar to natural testosterone.

The drug was initially manufactured to be used for veterinary purposes. It was used to increase the efficiency of race horses by enhancing their appetite and body muscles.

How the drug suddenly became popular amongst body builders is not known, but the drug is widely used by athletes due to its various advantages.

At a low dose, boldenone is a powerful anabolic agent, used to increase muscular mass when combined with a rich healthy diet.

However, at extremely high dose, the drug can have some pronounced side effects. It can lead to the suppression of natural testosterone production and hence leads to infertility. Further, inside the body, boldenone is converted into estrogen which causes gynecomastia in male.

Being anabolic in nature, the drug encourages protein synthesis and mineral nutrients balance within the body.

The drug has a well known effect of increasing the RBC (Red blood cell) count. This boost in RBCs results in an increase in the rate with which oxygen is carried to the body tissues.

Due to its long half life, the drug stays in the body for as long as a year.

Boldenone is known to have a slow and steady response. The drug takes its time, around 2-4 months, to show its effect. The up side is that the muscular weight gained is long lasting and not just water mass. It is pure muscular tissue.

The exact amount of high or low dosage was never defined for human use. However, experimentations show that 200—800 mg/week of boldenone is sufficient.

Having some androgenic properties, the drug has a number of side effects:

•	A change from normal to oily skin; this is due to the oily texture of this drug when injected.
•	Oily skin is more likely to have acne problems.
•	Hair loss is often witnessed in people on high drug dosage.
•	Like any other anabolic drug, boldenone causes mood swings, mainly resulting in aggression and depression.
•	Hypertension due to increase in metabolic rate.
•	Drowsiness and nausea.
•	Liver cancer may result due to the increased liver functioning.

Testosterone E

Testosterone E or Testosterone Enanthate is an artificial supply of the hormone testosterone.

The drug is taken normally to increase the level of testosterone in the body and is usually the first steroid prescribed by physicians for those with low Test E levels.

Testosterone E changes the appearance and size of the muscle tissues. Having androgenic properties, it protects the maintained build from getting broken down by the process of catabolism.

Testosterone works by stimulating the muscle cells to store more protein in the body. This protein is later used for enhancement of muscle fibers.

The effect of testosterone is further seen in causing an increase in the production of red blood cells in the liver. This raise in RBCs increases body's endurance and helps it to recover faster from any physical exertion.

Due to the powerful effects of this hormone, it should be taken once or at maximum, twice a month.

Body builders take advantage of the anabolic characteristics of testosterone E, and commonly inject a sufficient dosage of about 200-400mg/month.

The drug is usually taken off season as its half life is shorter than other anabolic drugs. The drug itself has slow response. It is often taken in combination with other drugs to enhance its effects and reduce the possible side effects.

A number of advantages of Testosterone E are:

- Makes the person healthy and fresh
- Enables the user to do more exercise
- Provides nutrient balance
- Increases muscular mass and results in fat loss
- Increases endurance level and body strength and patience
- Used to treat women breast cancer

The drug itself comes with a number of disadvantages as well. These include gynecomastia, hair loss, acne, deepening of voice, nausea, jaundice, liver malfunctioning, anxiety and depression.

To reduce the effects of gynecomastia, estrogen suppressant is taken along with testosterone E. This drug helps in removing the effect of estrogen produced, when a high dose of testosterone E is taken.

Special care should be taken by bodybuilders suffering from diabetes or having some cancer. It is not recommended for children, since it can cause puberty issues. For women, the drug can have adverse effects, like an increase in hair growth and deepening of voice. On the first sign of such effects, the drug should be immediately stopped.

Trenbolone A

Trenbolone acetate or Trenbolone A is a dream drug for bodybuilders. It is an anabolic drug which can either be injected or taken as pills. Claimed to be three times more powerful than testosterone, it does not get aromatized like other steroids.

Recommended dosage: Per day thirty five to seventy five milligram of Trenbolone should be consumed and this amount should be divided into two to four doses. For bodybuilders, the suggested quantity is seventy five milligram per day. It can be taken with or without meals.

Benefits of Trenbolone A: This drug is a very powerful androgen and has many benefits for bodybuilders;

•	Promotes muscle growth: It is the best drug for promoting muscle growth, strength and muscle mass. Users have experienced a "massive increase" in muscles in a quick time.
•	Ability to lean people out
•	Does not cause water bloating
•	Increase in strength
•	Hardens the body
•	Safe drug: As compared to other performance enhancing drugs Trenbolone A is much safer and has fewer side effects.
•	Promotes production of red blood cells
•	Enables quick recovery from injuries
•	Efficiency: It is said to give results quickly.

Trenbolone A Side Effects: For some people the side effects of this drug can be so harsh that they have to quit its use. Common side effects include:

•   Skin problems: It may cause redness, irritation, hives or swelling
•   Disturbed sleeping habits: Trenbolone acetate may influence the sleeping habits. It can even cause insomnia.
•   Cardiovascular problems: It causes high blood pressure which results in many cardiovascular diseases.

Nevertheless, many successful bodybuilders use this powerful drug despite its side effects just because it can enhance muscle strength significantly.

Primobolan

Primobolan is an injectable anabolic steroid which is usually used by bodybuilders for preparations. It is rather a weaker drug and consuming small amounts does not reveal any significant results.

Benefits of Primobolan: This drug is quite famous in bodybuilders and has certain benefits which no other drug offers;

•   Fat burning properties: Tests and experiments have revealed that Primobolan helps in reducing fat content of the body. It helps in weight loss and according to many bodybuilders they cannot even think about going on diets without Primobolan daily dosage.

- Increased muscle mass: Like many other steroids, Primobolan too helps enhance the muscle mass.
- No Aromatization: Primobolan does not convert into estrogen
- No water retention: As it does not aromatize, the side effects like water retention and acne don't occur with its use.
- Enhances immunity: Because of this property, Primobolan is said to be beneficial for AIDS patients too.
- Maintaining lean tissues: It helps gain and maintain more muscles while keeping the figure lean
- Nitrogen retention: It helps the body retain nitrogen. Nitrogen retention makes the body build more muscles.

Side Effects of Primobolan: Primobolan has milder side effects which disappear once its use is discontinued. Common side effects are:

- Hair loss
- Hormonal imbalance in women: It may cause an imbalance in women which results in deepening of voice, increase in body hair and irregular ovulation cycles.
- Hypertrophy in women
- Mild acne: In some cases the use of Primobolan results in mild acne on face, back and chest
- Increased aggression
- Insomnia

- Excessive sweating even while insignificant physical activity

Primobolan is generally accepted as a milder steroid and is most attractive among women owing to the fact that its side effects go away with treatments and discontinuation of the drug.

Testosterone P

When the male sex hormone known as testosterone is synthesized, it's appended to an ester in order to lag its release in the body. That shortest ester attached to testosterone hormone is known as Testosterone P.

Since Testosterone P has a very short term active life, therefore it's injected at least every other day unlike other anabolic steroids that are injected once in a week or once in every fifteen days.

Testosterone P is widely used by bodybuilders, weightlifters and other athletes for increasing muscle strength and boosting stamina. It is considered bodybuilder's favorite injectable steroid, as it provides a faster onset of progress.

This drug is often preferred over testosterone C and Testoveron Depot due to its less severe side effects, but one of its major side effects is its frequent schedule of dosage due to which a good number of people choose to stay completely away from this steroid.

But, those who are okay with repeating injections every other day find, this is really effective, as it's one of the most powerful mass building drugs available in the market.

It also boosts rapid increase in strength and muscle size and is also capable of reducing fats from the body.

One of its major positive effects is less water retention as unlike other anabolic steroids, its usage doesn't give a bloating and puffy look to the muscles.

Side effects of testosterone P include: Increased body and facial hair, oily skin, gynecomastia, aggression, prostate enlargement, and hair loss.

Testosterone C

Testosterone C or Testosterone Cypionate is one of the most prescribed types of testosterone mostly manufactured in USA.

When a body fails to generate the required testosterone, it results in abnormal conditions as sexual dysfunction, delayed puberty and lack of beard, pubic and chest hair. These conditions are treated through a process known as hypogonadism which usually involves the usage of testosterone C and various other anabolic steroids.

Testosterone C is creamy crystalline powder that is white in color, has almost no odor and is not dissolvable in water. Its chemical name is -4-en-3-one, 17-(3-cyclopentyl-1-oxopropoxy)-,

(17β)-. It is injected into the buttocks deep inside the gluteal muscle.

Testosterone C is commonly used by bodybuilders, weightlifters and other athletes around the world.

Some of its common side effects are: strokes, heart attacks, liver tumors, blood clotting in blood vessels, acne, cysts and oily skin and increased hair. Some abusers of testosterone C can also experience mood swings, irritability and aggressive behavior.

Testoveron Depot

Testoveron Depot is a multi-purpose steroid preferred by a number of athletes and body builders around the world in all degrees of training.

It's exceptionally effective for obtaining gigantic strength gains and developing amazing muscle weight. It's also useful in raising stamina and compressing the recovery time.

Testoveron Depot it's the most commonly used steroid for increasing strength, building muscles and losing fats.

Testosterone is responsible for the development of male sex organs and the insufficient production of testosterone results in psychic, anatomic and sexual deficiency in a person. Therefore, Testoveron Depot is considered an effective medicine for treating hypogonadism caused by the deficiency of androgen.

Bodybuilders call it "the mass building steroid" as it's the best way to increase muscle mass and strength with rapid weight gain. This drug is injected once in a week by weightlifters, bodybuilders, power lifters and other athletes.

While it has many positive effects, there are some side effects of Testoveron Depot as well, such as abnormal breast growth in men, puffy and bloated looking muscles, unwanted weight gain, impotency; acne on neck, shoulders and back; oily hair and skin, baldness, high blood pressure and liver impairment.

It is also said that when a person stops taking this drug, his strength and muscle mass start getting considerably reduced in a short span of time.

Chapter 10 Liver Protection

The intense amounts bodybuilding training with food, anabolic steroids and supplements can often take its toll on the liver.

A healthy liver is required for building muscles and losing extra fats as it's responsible for maintaining fats and protein transformation and refining the toxins in the body.

Bodybuilders are well aware of the importance of a healthy liver in the muscle building method; therefore, it's necessary that they maintain a healthy liver by taking few necessary precautions.

Oral steroids are very hard on the liver. Some bodybuilders and athletes take many drugs a day that can negatively impact their livers. Hence, injectable steroids are used by mainstream bodybuilders as they put less stress on the liver as compared to oral steroids.

Some painkillers i.e. Percocet, commonly used antibiotics, cholesterol medications and acetaminophen should not be used while on a cycle; they're liver killers.

Avoiding tobacco and alcohol is also a must for keeping a liver healthy. Other than that bodybuilders are also recommended to sleep well as the liver and immune system play the most important role in creating a synergistic effect.

Bodybuilders should also avoid taking lots of proteins in their daily diet. Protein intake above 350gms should be strictly avoided. Exercising can help in relieving stress and nurturing a healthy liver.

Some supplements that help in maintaining the liver in a good condition while on a cycle are: Milk thistle, NAC and Essentiale. Milk thistle is a common supplement for liver health.

NAC works by reducing the potency of bodybuilding steroids and protect the liver from detoxification.

Essentiale is used for the treatment of liver damage due to medicines or alcohol.

Bodybuilders are highly recommended to use these supplements while on their cycle; they're found to be the most effective liver health supplements today.

Chapter 11 Post Cycle Therapy

Post cycle therapy is essential to normalize the natural production of testosterone after a steroid cycle. For this purpose, athletes and bodybuilders make use of different drugs for post cycle therapy treatment which help restore testosterone levels or reduce estrogen levels.

The Use of Nolvadex

One of the most common types of drug used during PCT is a SERM (Selective Estrogen Receptor Modulator) which has the ability to inhibit estrogen production with respect to some genes and may also act as an estrogen with respect to others. One such SERM is Nolvadex which is commonly used by athletes and bodybuilders.

Nolvadex has estrogenic effects on bones, which brings about an increase in bone density making you stronger. It also prevents gynecomastia which is the abnormal production of mammary glands in males. Therefore, due to its discerning abilities towards some genes, such drugs are considered to be 'selective' in nature.

However, the use of Nolvadex in post cycle therapy treatment is not only because of its estrogen inhibition ability but also because it helps in raising testosterone levels in the human body.

Nolvadex has a special effect on the pituitary gland and hence the testosterone levels on the human body increase. On an average, 20 mgs of Nolvadex result in about 150% increase in testosterone levels.

Dosage of Nolvadex

Typically, doctors recommend 20 mgs of Nolvadex per day during PCT, yet, some may use higher doses. However, studies suggest a higher dose of Nolvadex or any other anti-estrogen for that matter is highly ineffective as it may not result in too much increase in testosterone levels. Therefore, doctors suggest that bodybuilders stack Nolvadex with other estrogen inhibitor drugs.

Drugs such as Arimidex or Letrozole might be used in small doses along with Nolvadex to prevent gynecomastia and increase testosterone production.

It is also useful to stack drugs for post cycle therapy treatment because you may not know what drug your body will respond to.

It also allows you to consume reasonable doses of each drug thereby preventing any negative effect demonstrated by consumption of large doses.

Clomid

Being a selective estrogen receptor modulator, clomid is a popular infertility drug in the medical world. But, owing to its property of blocking estrogen inhibition, it has exceptional benefits for bodybuilders and athletes.

Usually taken in the form of pills the generic drug in clomid is clomiphene citrate, a synthetic form of estrogen, which stimulates the production of testosterone. For this reason, it offers benefits for bodybuilders too. Although it is a weaker drug, it is used by many athletes to increase their testosterone levels and bind estrogen receptors. Athletes use it during post cycle therapy, for restoring natural testosterone levels in the body.

Clomid is weaker than nolvadex; 150 mg of clomid gives the same effect as achieved through using 20 mg nolvadex. However, the recommended per day dosage of clomid is around 50mg to 100mg.

Benefits of Clomid

- Stimulates release of testosterone
- Prevents gynecomastia

- Can be used safely as a long term treatment for low testosterone levels
- Has fewer side effects than other similar drugs such as nolvadex
- Normalizes hormone level in bodybuilders

Side Effects of Clomid

The side effects of clomid occur only if it is used in heavy doses for a long time.   Inappropriate doses also result in several negative side effects such as: vision problems, stomach ache, cardiovascular diseases, nausea; Including stomach ache, vomiting and severe feeling of nausea, headaches; prolong use of clomid results in headaches which can extend to migraines, stroke, chest pain, weight gain, back ache, hair loss, fatigue, dehydration of skin etc.

The drug is said to give positive results in most cases but should only be taken after proper consultation and expert advice.

The Use of HCG

Restoring endogenous testosterone production is of great concern at the end a steroid cycle. This is when low androgen levels lead to problems caused by negative feedback in the body due to synthetic steroid use.

The biggest concern is the action of cortisol, which in many ways is balanced out by the effect of androgens. Cortisol sends the opposite message to the muscles than testosterone, or to breakdown protein in the cell. Left unchecked (by an extremely low testosterone level) in the body, cortisol can quickly strip much of your new muscle mass away.

Human Chorionic Gonadotrophin, or HCG is a peptide hormone produced by the embryo during pregnancy and by placenta to help control hormones in pregnant women.

Bodybuilders use HCG for post cycle therapy because it mimics the Leutenizing Hormone which is what stimulates the testes to produce testosterone. HCG used during a cycle can help one avoid testicular atrophy. Some may still use HCG in reduced doses accompanied by drugs such as Nolvadex to deal with estrogen related side effects.

Chapter 12 Peptides

Peptide hormones are secreted by various endocrinal glands. They are synthesized by amino acids and are normally secreted directly to the blood stream. Being water soluble, peptide hormones take less time to start working as compared to steroid hormones which usually take a while to start functioning in the body.

Peptide hormones are also known as protein hormones and vary widely in size. Peptide hormones basically start the production of a large number of unique hormones which are essential for regulating important functions of human body. This is the basic reason why they are being commonly used by the bodybuilders to build more muscle.

To get to know more about peptide hormones, it is important to be aware of the various hormones constituted by the peptide hormones.

1.   ACTH (Adreno Corticotrophic Hormone):

This hormone is being secreted by the pituitary gland and helps in stimulating adrenal glands. It assists in administering the production of gluco-corticoids as well as growth hormone. It also helps in rebuilding the damaged tissues in the body and acts on muscles, bones and liver. Increased levels of this hormone can cause insomnia, hypertension and osteoporosis etc.

2.ADH (Anti Diuretic Hormone):

This peptide hormone aids the body in fluid retention and stimulates higher level of blood pressure.

3.HCG (Human Chorionic Gonadotrophic):

This hormone helps in increasing testosterone levels in the body. It can assure increased muscle mass and enhanced strength the body builders hanker after. However, an excessive level of even this hormone can cause a number of dreadful side effects. Among these side effects two of the most common and terrible ones are gynecomastia in males and disturbed menstrual cycle in females.

4.Luteneizing Hormone and Follicle Stimulating Hormone:

These hormones are produced by pituitary glands and stimulate gonads. They are responsible for building the secondary characteristics in males and females. Moreover, they help female bodies in maturation of ovarian follicles and play a vital role in production of sperms in males.

5.HGH (Human Growth hormones):

Human growth hormones are secreted by the pituitary gland in the human body and are responsible for the development of tissues and the breakdown of proteins and fats in the body.

As the name implies, these hormones are essential for administering growth of human body. It helps in increasing not just the size of the body cells but also the number of the cells. This hormone is among the most important hormones used by athletes for increasing muscle mass and enhancing strength.

However, an increased amount of HGH in body can make you suffer from a variety of disorders like hypertension, abnormal growth of hands and feet, increased perspiration, agitation etc.

Apart from these important peptide hormones, there are a number of others as well like EPO, (Erythropoietin) which is a hormone responsible for increasing the number of RBCs (Red Blood Cells) in human body and is normally considered to be effective for enhancing body endurance level. Some other vital peptide hormones are Gastrin, Prolactin, insulin etc.

Growth hormone is the fountain of youth and as one ages, body produces lesser amounts of growth hormone thus decreasing metabolism rate, muscle recovery, endurance and fitness.

Different variants of Growth hormone releasing peptides offer therapies that can help people in maintaining a steady flow of growth hormone by injecting these drugs to produce artificial stimuli that enhance secretion and production of growth hormone.

This enhanced production of growth hormone improves size and number of muscle cells, increases elasticity thus removing wrinkles, improves fitness, enhances testosterone levels and magnify endurance of the body. All these are attained with very minor or absolutely no side effects.

Bear in mind that some variants of Growth hormone releasing peptides are designed for professionals and they bring greater results but have many side effects associated with them. We are specifically talking about GHRP2, which brings enormous gains though they can't be compared to the gains brought by other drugs.

Growth hormone releasing peptides produce best results when taken under the supervision of doctors, knowing the right combination, dosage amount, frequency, training and rest pattern along with maintaining proper diet demands surveillance of a professional eye. All these factors are important in bringing the desired results.

After the age of 40, growth hormone is produced in very little quantities. This low level of growth hormone effects testosterone levels, causes the accumulation of body fats, and reduces rate of metabolism and hinders in maintaining blood sugar level.

HGH is generally stacked with other steroids for better results. Also, since most of the athletes have already reached their highest potential in deriving benefits from a specific steroid, small human growth hormone dosages along with other steroids help push the boundaries.

Due to its role in protein metabolism, HGH has found rapid usage by athletes and bodybuilders for muscle building purposes.

Bodybuilders and athletes usually prefer the use of HGH because it is considered to be safer, especially when taken in recommended

Older studies conducted on HGH dosages recommend 16.5 IU (international units) of HGH distributed in 3 doses during the week. However, such a dosage is considered to be high and is reported to increase the probability of side effects.

Modern physicians recommend lowered doses such as 4-8 IU every week distributed into 2 doses every day for a period of 6 days. Doctors also teach patients in injecting themselves with HGH early in the morning and at night. On the 7th day, HGH injections are not suggested.

Also, some doctors have been reported to prescribe very low HGH doses at the start such as 0.5 IU for a day. This dosage is gradually increased in an increment of 0.5 IU per month.
Side Effects

The side effects of HGH are believed to be visible with a dosage of 2 IU or higher. The most common side effect is the thickening of bones of forehead and hands, the enlargement of body organs like the heart and kidney and increased chances of hypoglycemia. The consumption of HGH is also believed to be linked with increased insulin resistance thereby resulting in diabetes in the user.

Global IGF-1

Insulin like growth factor, commonly known as Global IGF-1, is a performance enhancing experimental drug mostly used by bodybuilders. This drug directly affects muscles, cartilage bones, lungs, liver, nerves and skin. It is also found to have significant influence on cell development and growth.

Global IGF-1 is said to deliver the following benefits;

- Beneficial for health
- Helps in muscle growth
- Rejuvenates nerve cells
- Helps reduce fat and protein breakdown and makes protein transportation into cells easier
- Produces lymphocytes
- Reduces levels of bad cholesterol in the blood

As a result of weight training, new muscle cells are developed and this process is known as hypertrophy. When global IGF-1 is consumed, it helps in growth of muscle fibers by splitting muscle cells. This process is called hyperplasia. Hypertrophy combined with hyperplasia gives a new strength to muscles. Moreover, it also makes the recovery and repair of injured muscles quick. This is the reason this drug is getting popularity among bodybuilders. Although it is an experimental drug, yet the expectations from this drug are high.

Global IGF-1 is injected directly into the muscles and the best part about this drug is that it is undetectable by both urine test and blood test.

In a nutshell, this amazing drug provides perpetual muscle growth, anti-aging, and muscle repair without getting detected.

Glotropin

Glotropin is a human growth hormone which stimulates increased production of body's natural hormones like insulin. Its chemical composition includes about 191 amino acids bound together.

Glotropin has several advantages:

- Stimulates body cells to divide faster and grow in size
- Increases protein synthesis
- Increases muscular mass
- Enhances body's ability to use up fats and decreases carbohydrate breakdown. This is important, since carbohydrate storage in muscles needs to be maintained, if muscular body is required. Therefore, glotropin intake reduces body's fat deposition.
- Strengthens body tissues
- Provides faster recovery from injuries

Dosage of glotropin varies from person to person. The hormone may be taken daily or thrice a week. It all depends on your body size and weight.

Apart from the above mentioned advantages, like every steroid, glotropin has its bleak side as well:

- Bone deformations
- Improper functioning of thyroid gland
- Acne
- Liver malfunctioning due to excessive stimulation
- Head ache and nausea
- May give physical build, but it cannot give much internal body strength. Therefore, it is often stated that the effects of this hormone are merely for show and not internal
- Water Retention
- Unnatural hair growth

Insulin

Insulin is a hormone naturally produced by pancreas in human body. This hormone works to keep the blood glucose level within an acceptable range. Insulin works by converting excessive sugar in our blood into glycogen, and hence depositing it in muscle tissues. Therefore, increased secretion of insulin provides a favorable environment for muscle build up.

Mechanism: It is important to feed your body with sufficient amount of carbohydrates and proteins to avoid breakdown of your muscular storage. Researchers have deduced that after vigorous workout, human body is more likely to breakdown carbohydrates than fats to meet the increasing need of energy. To avoid muscular mass getting broken down, an insulin shot just after exercise will help your body retain its carbohydrate storage in the muscles and instead force it to break fats down to meet body demands.

Side effects of insulin:

- Improper dosage can lead to fat deposition in body muscles.
- Insulin injection can hinder the natural production of this hormone within our body. If this situation occurs, blood insulin level can increase. This will directly lead to diabetes.
- An increased level of insulin might result in a drastic reduction in blood glucose level. This can result in coma, brain damage or even death.
- Therefore, insulin is a useful hormone if used with care.

Chapter 13 Prohormones

Prohormone supplements are anabolic precursors that act as anabolic steroids and enhance the growth and development of muscles in the body. These supplements are generally used by weight trainers or body builders to enhance muscle mass.

Usually, prohormone supplements lack only one molecule to be equivalent to anabolic steroids. Once these supplements are digested, and the enzymatic process takes place, the missing molecule is introduced in the body resulting in an increase in the anabolic hormones in the blood stream. This facilitates a chemical reaction that helps to burn the extra body fat and nutrients and building muscle mass.

Due to the limited amount of enzymes available in the body, the result of prohormone supplements may be restricted. When the body gets short of the enzymes used to break down hormones, the performance of the supplements becomes reduced.

Androstenedione is a prohormone supplement which is an antecedent for testosterone. Similarly, DHEA or dehydroepiandrosterone is a precursor to many other hormones in the body and is typically used to increase athletic performance, enhance strength, support weight loss and also develop cognitive ability.

Some people may believe that the usage of prohormone supplements is extremely beneficial without any side effects, however, prolonged usage results is many side effects and various organ complications.

Excess use or misuse of prohormone supplements may result in liver complications. Moreover, prolonged use may also lead to renal failure and may also affect fertility in the long run. Extensive use causes hair loss, acne and baldness as it eventually lowers the production of testosterone in the body with the passage of time.

In females, the abuse of prohormones may lead to the development of masculine features such as increased facial growth or deepening of voice. This occurs due to the increase in testosterone production in women through the usage of prohormone supplements. Therefore, before taking any type of prohormone supplement, it is recommended to consult a doctor.

Considering these complications and the misuse of steroids and prohormones by many athletes, some prohormone compounds were banned under the Anabolic Steroid Control Act of 2004.

Recommended use of prohormones is after the age of thirty. People below twenty one should not even think about using them.

Prohormone Benefits

- Muscle growth: They help in increasing the muscle mass significantly and make the body look bigger.
- Muscle strength: Prohormones are popular for enhancing muscle strength.
- Appetite: Increased appetite is another benefit of using these supplements.
- Recovery time: In athletes, the use of prohormones enhances the recovery time.

Harmful Effects of Prohormones

The side effects of using prohormone usually vary with the prohormone used. There are a number of common harmful effects:

- Liver function: Prohormones are said to be stressful for the liver.
- Hair loss: Imbalance of these can result in irrecoverable hair loss.

- Bad cholesterol: An increase in blood cholesterol level may occur.
- Acne: This is a side effect common to most steroids and prohormones.
- High blood pressure: Problems like high blood pressure and hypertension may occur.

Chapter 14 Weight Loss Drugs

Weight loss i.e. reducing extra fats or body weight is important for living a healthy and controlled life. The methods used by bodybuilders for achieving their desired weight loss are: dieting, training, steroids and supplements. All these combined with enormous motivation result in an amazingly built body with no excessive fat.

Steroids help bodybuilders to maintain weight loss by repartitioning body fats. Various anabolic androgenic steroids aid in reducing excessive weight and increasing lean body mass. These steroids are also useful in building strong muscles and strengthening the stamina.

Bodybuilders also control their proteins and carbohydrates intake when they're on their weight loss cycle.

Training is the most important component of weight loss as it's great for burning calories. During bodybuilding training, the body is forced to utilize the stored fat which results in a good weight loss.

Weightlifting is also very helpful in this regard and bodybuilders can acquire a maintained and desirable physique by weightlifting 4 to 6 times a week. In addition to it, five to six cardio workouts every week for 30 minutes each can be really beneficial for losing excessive fats.

Cardio workouts include: biking, running and brisk walking etc.

Various supplements also aid in the phase of weight loss. Bodybuilders require supplements in order to meet their high protein needs. Protein powders are found pretty useful in this regard, as they are effective in attaining sufficient protein levels. There are some controversial supplements too which are not recommended to use as their side effects mostly overcome their benefits.

Clenbuterol

Clenbuterol drug is prescribed to the asthma patients as a treatment to the disease. More often, it is used to enhance weight loss or as a performance enhancement drug, mostly utilized by athletes and body builders. This drug is identified as sympathomimetics, which implies that it directly affects the nervous system to execute its performance enhancement function.

Clenbuterol directly affects the beta-2 sympathomimetics receptors along with the beta-1 receptors. These beta-1 receptors directly influence the cardio levels in such a way that it affects the body activity. Clenbuterol performs the same function as performed by epinephrine and generally affects the human body by carrying out the following actions:

- Stimulates the receptors in such a way that it enhances the aerobic activity of the body.
- Quickens the Central Nervous System of the human body.
- Increases the blood flow in the arteries thereby increases the blood pressure
- The transfer of oxygen is also enhanced
- Helps in enhancing the Body Mass Index of the body by efficiently increasing the metabolism rate of the body.
- At the same time it also helps in loosening up of the muscles.

As mentioned above, it increases metabolism rate thereby blood pressure goes high. This means that the body mass index is increased and at the same time body fats are burned due to increased blood activity.

The side effects of Clenbuterol includes: hypertension, hypersensitivity, acute myocardial infarction etc. Clenbuterol is banned in many States due to its harmful effects.

Cytomel T3

Cytomel T3 is a synthetic thyroid hormone, That is especially popular among body builders to burn fat. Cytomel T3 however is not directly produced by the thyroid; in fact it is converted into T4 hormone to carry out its function.

Cytomel T3 is a thyroid agent which directly affects the mitochondria, often referred to as the powerhouses of the cells, to perform its activity enhancement function. It stimulates mitochondria to increase the amount of ATP produced which in turn increases the production of energy in the human body. This means, respiration activity is increased to produce more heat in the body.

Following are some of the advantages of the drug:

- Enhances metabolism rate reducing weight effectively
- Helps in breaking down of proteins more efficiently to produce high energy
- Keeps a hormonal balance in the body
- Reduction of Goiter is an apparent affect of this drug

Body builders utilize Cytomel T3 because of its property of eradicating "sticky fats" from the body, thereby helping reduce weight, but not the body mass index, efficiently.

The starting dosage of Cytomel T3 must be low; 25mcgs per day is enough in the start which can gradually be increased as the days pass by.

Over dosage of this prescription is strictly prohibited. It should not be taken for more than five weeks after which it will start affecting the thyroid gland.

As this is an addictive drug, the dosage must be reduced gradually. Side effects of this Cytomel T3 include: headache, insomnia, diarrhea, sudden weight loss, fever, heat sensitivities and nervousness.

Xenical

Xenical is a drug prescribed to obese people which helps them lose all the extra fat from the body. This weight losing drug is especially prescribed to people having health issues like diabetes, blood pressure or high cholesterol.

Xenical is however most popular amongst the body builders who take this drug as a dietary supplement along with their workout routine.

The main function of this supplement is to absorb the fats and keep away from accumulating inside the body. This drug is basically a gastrointestinal lipase inhibitor which prohibits the fats from settling inside the body, with an absorption rate of thirty percent.

When taken along with hard core exercise and a low fat routine, this prescription is reported to give the best results.

Before using this drug, it is advised to consult a medical practitioner to avoid any kind of complications. However, as a general pattern, it is taken one hour after the consumption of a meal containing fats. Body builders are advised to take it three times a day as their supplement routine.

Following are some of the apparent advantages of using Xenical:

* Reduces weight up to 10% which is the reason why it is one of the most recommended drugs for body builders.
* Helps in lowering blood pressure and the sugar level.
* It is perfectly healthy for the digestive system with no side effects on cardiovascular system
* This drug is non-addictive.
* Tolerability level of this prescription is also high.

Xenical comes with many side effects which include: stomach pain, diarrhea, nausea, rectal pain or sometimes loss of appetite. Other complications include fever, chills or even flu. Teeth problems are also expected along with minor skin rashes. Those who are already on other drugs like insulin or Neprol should also consult with the physician to confirm the compatibility of the medications with this drug. Only those who are above 18 are eligible to take Xenical.

Reductil

Commonly known as sibutramine, reductil is considered highly effective in treating obesity. This drug works in two productive ways; first it builds a feeling of fullness so that the patient feels satisfied in a flash even after an intake of little portions of meal and it also reduces the frequency of cravings for unhealthy food. Secondly, it aids in restraining the metabolism of the body from slowing down.

The most active ingredient found in reductil is sibutramine hydrochloride monohydrate which is considered efficacious for reducing weight. The working of reductil is different from traditional weight loss pills as it operates by obstructing the re-uptake of a neurotransmitter known as serotonin. It results in the presence of a greater quantity of serotonin in the brain that is linked with smaller appetite.

Reductil is found in five, ten and fifteen milligrams doses and is only taken orally. It is mostly recommended to people who have tried different weight loss methods but nothing worked and having body mass index BMI of over 30 kg/m^2. Not every person using reductil report side effects but some of its common side effects are: nausea, hot flushes, headache, insomnia, constipation, sweaty hands and dry mouth etc. This drug is not considered an addictive medicine as it is licensed to use for long durations for treating obesity.

Sibutramine

Sibutramine, a medicine which has been withdrawn from the U.S and other regions market from October 2010, was primarily used to assist overweight people in losing weight by adjusting neurotransmitters inside the brain.

Neurotransmitters are defined as chemicals generated and released through nerves for communicating with other nerves. The neurotransmitters released may stick to other nerves or may be absorbed again by those nerves that usually release them. This processed is called reuptake. Thus, sibutramine used to obstruct reuptake of serotonin, norepinephrine and neurotransmitters dopamine. This obstruction of the reuptake of neurotransmitters alters neurotransmitters balance inside the nerve cells which affects the interaction and function of the nerve.

Sibutramine belongs to the "appetite suppressants" class of medications that help in reducing the cravings and hunger through alteration in the appetite control centers present in the brain.

Sibutramine was considered an effective drug for weight loss when taken with a healthy low calorie diet and exercise. It was also recommended for treating obesity related to high cholesterol, diabetes and high blood pressure.

This medicine was not commonly prescribed and people suffering from anorexia nervosa were not allowed to take it. Bodybuilders who used to take sibutramine were likely to achieve a reduction of 5 to 10% from their weight.

The reason of its withdrawal was some of its side effects that were found potentially hazardous and life threatening.

Diaretics

Diaretics also called water pills are medications that expel fluids from the body by increasing urination. Bodybuilders who need to cut down more weight in a short span of time turn to diaretics as the less fluid they have in their body, the less they will weight, and also more muscle definition.

There are several categories of diaretics but all of them work more or less differently. Major over the counter diaretics work on the kidneys for expelling salts and water. Other water pills increase blood supply to the kidneys and some drugs increase the filtration rate of the kidneys.

Diaretics is also used for treating conditions such as high blood pressure, kidney diseases, heart failure and liver cyrrohsis, but it is being advertised more as a weight reducing drug to normal users.

Diaretics is not considered a healthy way to reduce weight, as it is not proven to help in the fat reduction. This drug only aids in reducing the amount of liquid retained in the body. This weight loss is temporary and as soon as a user eats or drinks something, his body starts replacing the lost liquids, which results in a regain in his weight.

Other than that abusing diaretics may result into life threatening conditions like dehydration and critical potassium deficiencies. Moreover, some users also experience cramping or weakness of muscles, irregular heartbeat, fatigue and nausea.

Chapter 15 Underground Labs

Because steroids have been more difficult to get underground labs have sprung up all over the world to meet the demand. Because underground labs do not have to meet the stringent standards, required by legitimate pharmaceutical companies the quality may vary from batch to batch.

Because of the lack of quality control underground labs can be a dangerous choice. There have been reports of heavy metals, and other contaminants in all kinds of drugs from underground labs.

Generally speaking most products from underground labs are as safe as one made from legitimate pharmaceutical companies. You do have to be careful though; finding legitimate underground sources can be challenging.

Its a well known fact that steriods, and other drugs such as HCG, HGH, Viagra, and many, many other drugs can be purchased online; however, most suppliers that advertise online will not supply you with steroids at all. Most of them will take your money and you will never hear from them again.

The safest way to find a supplier is through the

recommendation of a friend, or through a networking group of bodybuilders.

There are free networking sites where you can find sources, but free is not always the best choice. Most free sites are sponsored and therefore the reviews may be moderated, and unfavorable reviews removed. Because of this a paid source check site is your best bet.

With a paid source check site you get reviews from people who buy online and take the whole matter very seriously. There are no sponsors, and reviews are not moderated.

Recommended Resources:

http://www.legitsteroidwebsites.com/: Free to join. Excellent forum. Sources are top-notch.

http://www.sourcecheckgroup.com/: Paid membership required.

Lots of sources, many that cannot be found anywhere else.

Chapter 16 Basics Of Nutrition

Steroid usage needs to be supplemented with a good and nutritious diet. In this chapter we would be taking a closer look at what exactly qualifies as nutritious. There are certain characteristics and ground rules that define a diet comprising of the right nutrition values. Play and fiddle around with these rules till the time you are sure of what kind of diet suits your needs the most. You can then make your own diet routines and list down your own diet plans.

Maintaining the balance:

Proteins, carbohydrates and fat are the three major constructs of a balanced diet. Other things like fiber, minerals and fluids also play an important role. Proteins help in bulking up. They are the building blocks of the body. Carbohydrates help in increasing the sugar levels of the body- thus providing adequate energy for the body to expend on working out. Fat keeps the muscles and the bones lubricated apart from providing the heart with healthy cholesterol and also helping to maintain the overall stature of the body. Thus, you meal can be tweaked to the kind of workout you intend to indulge yourself in. If you are doing heavy weightlifting then you can increase the protein intake and keep the other two variables constant. If you are looking to loose weight, then lowering the carbohydrate intake can really do wonders. If you are looking to loose out on body fat, then say no to greasy food items. You should, however, not cut down on any one of the three main constituents all at once. Doing so might fetch you fast results, but it'll hamper the overall equilibrium of your body. The ideal ration should be 40% each of proteins and carbs and 20% of fat, fiber and other minerals. The equation can be further simplified by having the same serving of proteins for an equivalent serving of carbs- plus stuff like green vegetables, fruits and milk to cover up for the other elements of a balanced diet.

Time your calories:

Calorie timing is a relatively new concept, but it is designed to prevent the plateau from occurring. Calories should be properly cycled as this prevents the body and the metabolism from getting used to a particular amount of calorie intake- thus leading to stagnant results. For those looking to gain muscle mass, you should stick to 5 days a week of heavy calorie intake (lean mass) and 2 days of low intake. For those looking to reduce body fat, you should focus on 5 days of low calorie intake and two days of high intake. For those who are looking to build muscle while loosing body fat, should randomize things up even further. For those who are looking to tone their bodies without really worrying about the muscle mass or the body fat percentage- you can switch between high and low calorie diets every week. This will keep your metabolism from stabilizing at lower levels.

Number of meals a day matters a lot:

It is a popular practice amongst bodybuilders to have six or eight smaller meals spread equally throughout the day rather than having two or three larger meals. This not only helps in keeping the body nourished all through the day, but it also helps in ensuring that if you are doing heavy workout, you do not fall short of body sugar and energy levels. This is one of the easiest ways of maintaining a healthy diet while working out.

Chapter 17
What Are Carbohydrates, proteins and fats, and How Do They Effect Me?

Carbohydrates:

Carbohydrates are the primary source of natural energy for the human body. Insulin is produced by the body when the pancreas burn carbs and insulin is elementary for the body since it helps the body in getting the much needed energy. Insulin breaks carbs into suitable substitutes and stores them either as fat or in the muscles. The storage is dependent upon how one utilizes the energy derived from carbohydrates. Insulin also helps in grabbing proteins (amino acids) and helps in storing the amino acids inside the muscle cells. This not only helps in growth, but also helps in recovery of the fatigued muscles. Therefore, insulin plays a major role in muscle building and the production of insulin is directly triggered by ingestion of carbohydrates in the body.

Although carbohydrates are important for insulin production, yet a high carb diet may lead to excess insulin being produced, which in turn leads the body into storing every part of your diet as fat. More the insulin, more your body tends to get fatter. Lower insulin levels on the other hand might result in your body not being able to utilize the amino acids for proper growth.   Thus, the right amount of carb intake is elementary for a proportionate body building.

Carbohydrates are broadly classified into two types- simple carbs and complex carbs.   Complex carbs are relatively more difficult to break down and take time to be broken down thus, giving timed energy.   Simple carbs give immediate energy as they are easier to break down.   Normal meals should mainly consist of complex carbs but breakfast and post-workout meals should have an abundance of simple carbs.   The reason is simple- when the body is depleted of energy (in the morning or post workout), it requires instant energy to rebuild its internal glycogen levels and therefore, you should always stick with simple carbs.   Complex carbs should be thrown out proportionately during the meals in order to give your body a sustained and prolonged energy boost throughout the day.

Complex carbohydrates include starchy edible stuff like potatoes, rice, wheat flour etc. and some green vegetables. Simple carbohydrates consist of fruits like apples, bananas and orange.   Mix and match the quantities to suit your body's needs and your workout timings.

Proteins:

Even if you are a beginner at bodybuilding, you would have definitely heard a lot about proteins and how they are the building blocks of the body. The fact remains that each and every tissue of the human body is made up of proteins and therefore, if you are looking to increase lean muscle mass- you ought to increase the protein intake in your day to day meals. Having said that, it is not as simple as it sounds. Proteins and carbs work in tandem. Carbs give the body the energy to convert protein into muscle while proteins help in the timing of carbs- thus providing all throughout the day. Besides, having proteins increases the metabolism of the body by up to 15% at a time and this is a very significant figure for those looking to burn fat and increase lean muscle mass.

The equation for protein consumption is simple. For every pound of your weight, you should consume 1 to 1.5 grams of protein. For instance, if you weight 200 pounds, you should consume about 175 grams of protein everyday. More than that might get converted into fat and lower protein levels will not give optimal results. Therefore, measuring and timing are the two most important aspects of maintaining a balanced protein diet. As a thumb rule, you should consume an equitable amount of carbs as well- this aids in protein synthesis.

Remember- carbs and proteins should always work in tandem rather than contradicting each others' effects on the human body. Eggs, chicken, turkey, fish and bacon are good examples of proteins.   Mix and match with other meat types to get the required amount.

Fats:

This is where it gets tricky.   The main purpose of a bodybuilding diet is to increase muscle.   Some people have a notion that the best way of doing it is by reducing the fat intake- and this notion, our dear readers, it dangerously convoluted!

Fats aid in hormonal reactions, they help in keeping the joint lubricated and their absence makes the body look out for fats. This will results in all of the food you consume to be accumulated as fat, which would hamper testosterone production in the body- thereby hampering the whole process of muscle building.   You might end up loosing weight and this will be counter productive to your over all bodybuilding regimen.   Therefore, in order to have a balanced metabolism running, you should always look towards including healthy fats in your diet. Fats are broadly classified into three types- saturated, monosaturated and polysaturated.

Saturated fats are the primary culprits behind heart related diseases, including high cholesterol levels and heart attacks. Saturated fats are found mostly in red meat and hydrogenated vegetable oils- mainly constituting packaged food. If there is something you really need to avoid when it comes to fats- its saturated fats.

Polysaturated fats have no effect on body cholesterol levels and are therefore the better of the three types of fats. These are mostly found in vegetable oils that do no get hydrogenated to saturated fats. Common examples include sunflower, soybean and cottonseed oil.

The best of the three fat varieties is monosaturated fats. These fats help in increasing the levels of "good" cholesterol in the human body. These might have antioxidant properties as well- something that really aids in establishing a healthy metabolic rate. When combined with protein shakes and carbohydrates (like wheat bread) monosaturated fats can really give your cardiovascular system a positive boost up. Some common sources of monosaturated fats include fish, flaxseed oil, olive oil and peanut butter.